Eati

For Busy Adults

By Joe Hashey

Dedication

Thank you to my family for their never ending patience. I truly appreciate it Melanie, Logan, Henry, and Everett.

This book was written for our amazing members at Synergy.

Thank you for trusting us with your fitness!

I received a lot of help from our staff along the way, especially Christa Reese.

I hope you enjoy and find value in reading it!

Preface

After a decade of owning and operating fitness studios, I've seen the struggle over nutrition first hand.

After all, an hour workout session is such a small portion of the day. Members would then be faced with free goodies at work, a standoff with the snack cupboard, and kids that prefer unhealthy food for dinner.

They'd get on Google and talk to their friends to find out what they were doing.

One person would recommend Keto.

Another co-worker would insist on Paleo.

A third colleague would have a shake a day plan.

Either the member would freeze due to too much information or half heartedly start a plan knowing that most fail. A few weeks or a month later it would be back to the drawing board.

This cycle is completely understandable with respect to all the obstacles.

There's the allure of the fast weight loss plans, the struggle of making it work as a busy adult, and feeling overwhelmed by everything else to manage in life.

It almost seems like too much to ever handle!

"Eating Strategies for Busy Adults" will provide clarity within the foggy world of diets and eating plans.

Instead of focusing on flashy tips that get minimal long term results, you'll learn the big picture strategy that you can apply right away.

Why trust me?

We've been fortunate enough to have access to one of the busiest InBody composition analyzers in the country. Each month we have hundreds of members track their eating and test their results.

The InBody is a medical grade body composition analyzer (think of a super fancy scale) that tells us if the person is losing weight, gaining muscle, adding water or any combo of the above.

We hear their feedback, watch their results, and discuss their habits - year after year, over and over again.

All the data and feedback has been eye opening.

It hasn't been "one plan" that created all the successes. It was an overall strategy that the members successfully implemented, often without realizing it!

I have nothing to sell you. No multi-level marking supplement plan, no diet cookbook or meal delivery service. Even as I write the book, the plan is to give away the first 1,000 copies to members completely at our cost.

I know that sharing this strategy will help guide our members towards their goals. By putting this in their hands, they'll reach their goals faster than ever and tell their friends.

My incentive is to set you up with a remarkable book to help guide you for years to come. That way, if you happen to live by one of our Synergy locations, you'll visit with the confidence that we have your back.

What this book is...and isn't.

This book is written to simplify and demystify your eating life. It will explain a new concept we use called '"eating profiles" and help you select the one that is the best fit for YOU.

Your profile will act like a key to unlock which diet plan or plans will work based on your activity level, mindset, and eating preferences.

There's a lot of marketing around flashy pictures, tips and tricks. Just last week I was standing in line at Wegmans and saw a magazine with a big headline stating "One Trick To Drop 20 lbs." I couldn't help but flip open to that page. It was a three page ad for Apple Cider Vinegar.

These flashy headlines are designed to catch your eye and can actually be helpful tiny pieces in a huge puzzle. But if you only implemented that one suggestion, nothing would really change.

Instead, we're going to step back, lay out all the pieces, and set you up to complete the "puzzle" as it is suited for your lifestyle.

This book is not an overly complicated in-depth scientific discussion. I will intentionally avoid the science-y jargon often used to create confusion. Also, if you're looking for a disease specific approach, then I'd highly recommend having a sit down with a good nutritionist.

In other words, if you're a professional bodybuilder looking to break down your micro and macro nutrients around competition season, this book will not be a great fit.

However, if you're a busy adult looking to renew your energy and feel like you're fully in control of your eating plan, then you'll want to read on.

Reading and taking action on these strategies may just change your life.

Section One - Developing A Game Plan

It's like learning to ride a bike

My older brother Don peered over the handlebars of his tiny Huffy bicycle and saw nothing but blue sky straight ahead.

Glancing downward, he saw the Catherine Street hill. It was a doozy of a hill directly outside our tiny house in Bangor, Maine.

Nerves took the better of him and he started to breathe fast.

He started to get cold feet and wanted off the bike.

Still my father guided him upright and gave him a gentle push.

Over the course of the next hour, there were tears, arguing, and a few scraped knees. Despite the difficulty and struggle, Don had learned to ride a bicycle in less than an hour and grew to love it.

Two years later it was my turn. My mother didn't really condone the "push them down the road" method of learning how to ride a bike fast. It was too aggressive.

I was peering over the handlebars at a large grassy slope at the former George H. Nichols elementary school in Endicott, New York.

After a "gentle" push I made it about 10 feet and fell over. The grass was a much softer fall but also bumpier. The bumps made it more challenging for a first time bike rider to stay upright.

It took all weekend until I could stay upright down the hill and across the field. It was a much longer time, still had its tearful moments, but at the end of the weekend I could ride my bike.

Both of my younger brothers received the standard training wheels. They rode for months with the little wheels holding them upright until it was time to take them off and go on their own.

It was a much slower process, but today they too can ride a bike well.

So which method was right?

All of us learned to ride at a different speed.

All of us know how to ride bikes.

All of the methods worked.

The same is true for healthy eating strategies. We spend hours laboring over which diet or eating plan is the #1 best of all times.

The truth is that the majority of the diets WILL work.

They use the same underlying principles which we will discuss more in depth shortly.

Eating plans should not be looked at like they are a multiple choice question on the SATs with one right answer and the rest are wrong.

Instead, they are more like an open ended essay question that you can answer based on your experiences, tastes, and preferences.

Once you understand this concept, it will open up a whole world of stress-free healthy eating choices to best fit your busy life.

Right Questions, Wrong Time

Should I eat fruit?

What should I have before my workout?

What's the best breakfast?

Should I eat almonds or peanuts?

Is _____ an okay meal to have?

Questions like this are great, however, they shouldn't be our first thought. These are tactical questions and are perfect to ask AFTER you choose your strategy.

Imagine a professional football coach being asked, "Should we run the ball?" It's a near impossible question to correctly answer without knowing more about the strategy.

Is it the 4th quarter with a lead?

Is it the 4th quarter and you're losing?

What plays have worked in the past?

The coach will need to understand the strategy of the game before calling individual plays.

As we prepare to dive into the eating profiles, keep in mind that these are the big picture strategies that you'll be able to apply when answering the majority of your tactical questions.

Just because you can, doesn't mean you should

An important footnote before we get into the exciting new information:

The eating profiles you're about to learn will provide clarity on an overall eating strategy that will not only be useful for weight loss, but also for renewing your energy and feeling great.

Although the eating profile terminology is new, it's the same overall approach that has worked for hundreds of our clients.

You *can* lose weight or structure your eating in other ways.

There was a trainer a few years back that lost weight on a fast food diet.

Another ate only potatoes for a month.

A third didn't eat for 60 days.

Just because you *can* use extreme methods doesn't mean you should. There are other factors that matter A LOT besides just weight loss.

You could eat only two Snickers bars a day and probably lose weight. Your energy levels will be all over the place, you'll be short on important nutrients, and you'll feel like crap, but you'd at least lose weight.

I wouldn't consider that an optimal, or even practical, approach.

This is important to keep in mind when the next extreme diet trend rolls around and you start hearing about it from a co-worker.

Classic Fable of the Tortoise and the Hare.

The tortoise moved so slowly that a hare began to mock him and ask, "Do you ever get anywhere?"

Due to the rabbit's arrogant behavior, the tortoise challenged him to a race.

The distance was marked off and the spectators gathered.

Right from the beginning, the hare ran out of sight.

To embarrass the tortoise, the rabbit decided to lay down and take a nap to prove that he could win in his sleep.

While the hare napped, the tortoise crept by him with a slow and steady pace.

The rabbit awoke to see the tortoise approaching the finish line!

He began to sprint, but could not overtake the tortoise.

Aesop's moral of the story was that "The race is not always to the swift."

Turtles, Rabbits, Spectators and Eating

Managing expectations and goals is one of the most critical steps to setting up a plan. Let's apply this story to what we see happen with fitness and nutrition.

Rabbits

The rabbit sprinted out fast like those on the restrictive eating plans. They'll often lose the first 5-10 lbs quickly. Eventually they'll lose focus or willpower to stick to the plan and fall back into old habits.

Turtles

The turtle in the fable had a slow and steady game plan and stuck to it. The same can work in the kitchen to allow leeway within a busy lifestyle.

Unfortunately, we're not always so lucky with eating. Often turtles will see the rabbit's quick success, become frustrated, and fall into unhealthy habits.

Baby Turtles

Not mentioned in the fable is the next generation of racers. Inspired by their parents' success in the "great race," they also want to try their luck. They begin setting up healthy habits like going for walks and getting a good night's sleep.

They're much more fragile and can be knocked off course by others' opinions, a few busy days, or confusion over what to do.

Spectators

Then there are those that gather to watch the race. They enjoy watching from the sidelines and admire the accomplishments of those competing.

However, they don't think that they could ever do it personally and don't even know where to get started. Although we'll provide lists of specific habits for rabbits, turtles, and baby turtles, spectators need more support to get started. If you identify yourself as a spectator, this is an important first step to get the ball rolling.

Moral

Each profile above has the opportunity to succeed and there is no one "right" way to run the race.

If rabbits have a plan to bridge back to practical eating after a sprint period, then they can be very successful.

If turtles set the right expectations and view their plan as a practical long term strategy, then they'll reach their goals.

If the baby turtles can filter through the flashy marketing messages and stay the course, they too will start to feel better and get more energy.

If the spectators can use the motivation to start thinking about their health, an important awareness will occur and they will start to seek guidance.

This needs to be said again. There is no RIGHT way to run this race. Even in Aesop's fable, both the tortoise and hare pass the finish line, and nearly at the same time.

Now that we have laid out the big picture, let's break down each profile into habits and actionable steps.

You can then choose the best fit and get in the race!

Your Eating Profile Task

As you read the following profiles, identify which one you fit into now.

Understand that you can switch profiles easily week to week (and probably should)!

For now, let's find your starting point.

Eating Profile #1: Rabbit

The rabbit is for someone that is going "all in." It's the most strict approach.

Characteristics of a rabbit:

- Focus on fast weight loss

- Meals consist mostly of lean meats, nuts, eggs, and veggies

- Commit to a 3-4 day a week fitness plan with added non-gym exercise

- Prioritize losing weight over getting stronger

- Cut out alcohol

- Typically motivated by a challenge or date (like a wedding)

- Typically sustainable for 3-8 weeks.

Strengths: Fastest weight loss with clear and structured eating rules.

Weaknesses: Rebound weight gain if there is no deeper reason "why" to continue after the challenge or date has passed. There needs to be a bridge program back to sustainable eating. Rigid rules make it difficult for an adult with a family.

Most of those probably make sense except for the "prioritize losing weight over getting stronger."

We've seen the data on our InBody over and over. Beginners to fitness can both lose fat and gain lean muscle since they haven't worked out before.

Over time, it becomes near impossible to both restrict calories for weight loss and to have a surplus for muscle gain at the same time. Setting this exception is critical.

Rabbits can't have it all. Their weight loss will come first over feeling full of energy during exercise. You can limit this weakness by focusing on the big picture exercises, taking full rest time, and getting a good night's sleep.

Big 5 Rabbit Habits

Simplifying all this information is the challenge. However, to make it actionable, it needs to be easily understood.

For our members looking to do a "rabbit sprint," we'll do daily check ins on the following 5 habits. This isn't an all inclusive list, but is enough to keep you on track for your results.

Rabbit Habits

1. Vegetables with every meal

2. Lean protein source with every meal

3. No alcohol

4. 60 minutes of exercise or activity

5. Full night's sleep

Some might be surprised by the sleep requirement. Sleep is when your body rebuilds. If you're not turning off the streaming video and hitting your pillow on time, you're not going to get great results. Plus, you'll likely burn out a lot faster. You'll need around 8 hours for best results.

As a quick note, when you change your eating, your sleep patterns will change. Often you'll have more energy and need to be purposeful about getting your sleep habits back in alignment.

The rabbit habits are the most strict. There's no "kind of" or "sort of" eating healthy. If your goal is to follow a strict plan, that means you have to check all the boxes.

If you're not 5/5, you're likely in the turtle profile up next.

Eating Profile #2: Turtle

The turtle profile is for someone that is following great habits most of the time.

Characteristics of a Turtle

- Exercises 3-4 days a week

- Follows the 80/20 rule in the kitchen. 80% of meals are healthy and they allow 1-2 "cheat" meals per week

- Plans meals around social gatherings to allow themselves to enjoy the gathering

- Plans days around the cheat meal to consume less or exercise more

- Quickly rebounds by not stringing cheat meals together.

- Does not turn a cheat meal into a cheat day and then into a cheat weekend.

- Most meals have a veggie and a protein

- Limits alcohol around their 80/20 rule

- Puts their carb/energy intake around their workout sessions

- Has a meal plan that includes family members. Does not wander into the kitchen and ask "Hmm, what should I eat now?"

Strengths: Balanced plan irons out too many ups and downs. Practical for families.

Weakness: Turtles often *think* they are rabbits and get frustrated with slower results. In other words, they've gone from no eating plan to this balanced approach but expect lightning fast results on the scale. If it doesn't happen fast, it knocks them off course easily.

Cheat meals roll into cheat days and there can be a constant cycle of being on/off track.

Last week I received an email that sounded like many others in the past.

"I need to share that I'm feeling frustrated. I've changed my eating, been to the workouts, and I'm only down 2 lbs!"

She was on her 11th day and had done 3 workouts.

I don't include this to make light of the situation. I've seen this many times before.

This is entirely my fault for not resetting her expectations first. After all, she's likely been swarmed with quick weight loss stories from magazines, social media, and co-workers. She doesn't know what to believe or trust.

Situations like these are the exact reason I'm writing this book. When you're empowered with real knowledge and expectations, you can navigate over these speed bumps.

Weaknesses: Frustrated by feeling like they have no control over family meals. Can easily fall off track if not supported. Can be tricked by clever marketing.

I had a former co-worker that insisted she was eating healthy. She read that low carbs will melt the fat away. The next day she had two dozen chicken wings for lunch because they were low in carbohydrates. She did not lose any weight.

Another was a new gym member that was having issues with weight loss so I asked for his food journal. After a quick review a few things stood out, like pizza for lunch and brownies with dinner. He explained that he used to have pizza with pepperoni and now he has it without for lower calories.

He was in the game, open to suggestions, and we looked at this as a mindset shift first. Eventually it clicked and he dropped the 20 lbs he had hoped.

Big 5 Baby Turtle Habits

1. Chews slowly to allow his/her body to feel full

2. Eats at least 1 vegetable a day

3. Focuses on replacing before restricting*

4. Exercises at least twice a week and is active outside workouts

5. Gets a full night's sleep most of the time.

*Replacing before restricting is an important concept that will be discussed more in depth in the frequently asked questions section. Essentially, you're not calorie counting. You're simply taking the unhealthy food you currently eat and replacing it with near the same quantity of healthy food.

With a baby turtle, there is a lot less focus on quick results. This can be a very freeing mindset for someone starting out!

They'll start to naturally move towards their goals by being more mindful of their choices.

The priority is to get momentum going with do-able steps and to avoid frustration. A big mistake would be to adopt these habits and weigh in every day and expect jaw dropping results.

Instead, focus on the mindful habit building process to make it stick.

If they have an expectation that it will be a slow process, baby turtles can be extremely successful in improving their long term health.

Eating Profile #4: Spectator

The legendary rabbit and turtle race must have gathered a crowd! The same goes for health and fitness stories.

Spectator Characteristics

- Busy with day to day life and eats what is around

- Paralysis by over analysis when it comes to eating plans

- No plan around fitness

- No plan around eating

- Frustrated by how they feel and not sure what to do about it

- Looking to get started "tomorrow," but tomorrow never seems to come.

- Aware but not active

Strengths: Still conscious of their overall health. Teetering on the fence and can be tipped into action with a practical plan.

Weaknesses: Frustration or embarrassment makes them weary of starting.

Spectators are often short a support system or guidance. If they had one or the other that was a fit for their style, they'd be willing to start their journey.

Big 5 Spectator Habits

1. Starts and stops healthy attempts from day to day

2. Eats whatever they have around

3. Confused by all the choices so chooses nothing

4. Avoids health conversations due to embarrassment

5. Does not think about sleep habits

If you find yourself in the spectator profile, there will be lots of actionable info in this book to help you get started. You don't have to choose it all. Pick 1-2 habits from any other profile that work for you and start there.

Which profile is best?

The best profile is the one that is currently most practical for you.

If you have a newborn and/or young children, you can slide into the turtle or baby turtle best. The rabbit profile would be the worst choice because sleep will be largely out of your hands and will only add to your stress.

If you grew up on PB&J and don't have a large recipe variety that includes vegetables yet, start with a baby turtle and build up. Otherwise your will power will get exhausted too quickly.

If you're doing wedding prep and have a few extra pounds to shed in a hurry, then you'll need to leverage the rabbit profile.

Best Practices and Action Steps

You're not married to one profile forever. A successful strategy is to choose the one that fits your goals and is practical right now.

Next, lay out a calendar for the year.

Look at holidays, birthdays, and major events.

Write down which profile you plan on following based on this information.

For example, Thanksgiving to end of January contains a lot of family get togethers, holidays, and birthdays for me.

I'll slide into the turtle habits to make sure I don't get off the rails between events. Next, I'll plan more challenging training sessions to use the calorie surplus to gain lean muscle and boost metabolism.

When February comes around, it's time for a change to rabbit mode until my birthday on March 25th.

After that we'll go back to turtle through the summer. The fall is my second "rabbit" season and I'll dial it in until Thanksgiving.

Every month has an overall profile that is practical to follow. For me, in a calendar year it's only realistic to spend a total of 8-10 weeks in the rabbit profile.

Setting a full plan with beginning and end dates makes it easy to follow the strict guidelines when I've decided to implement them.

For you, there may be a lot of summer travel. Use that time to back off BUT still have a plan. (Don't toss it all out!)

If you think ahead and write down the year's gameplan, you'll be light years ahead.

Why Diets Work

Popular diets work because of the same underlying principles. They limit your choices and therefore limit the calories you consume overall.

I'm NOT suggesting this is a bad thing.

Instead, it should be freeing.

The plans below can certainly work for you if it's a fit for your busy life. Many of them will fit the rabbit profile and you can use them to reach your goals.

You'll know that after you choose your eating strategy, you can choose whichever diet fits your unique tastes and preferences. Plus you won't be married to one plan and burn out. You can rotate seasonally based on the produce you like to purchase or even simply to get a change.

Here's a list and a quick overview of how the diet works to get you thinking. If you find one that seems like a fit for you, I'd suggest doing a little more research before diving in!

Whole 30 - Limits your calorie intake by limiting choices to whole single ingredient food.

Paleo - Limits your calorie intake by limiting choices to foods presumed to have been available during the Paleolithic era.

Keto - Limits your calorie intake by limiting choices to mostly fats.

Atkins - Limits your calorie intake by limiting choices to mostly proteins and staying low carb.

Vegetarian - Limits your calorie intake by limiting choices to plant or plant-based foods.

Fast Diet or 5:2 - Limits your calorie intake by limiting calories to ~500 on 2 days per week.

Intermittent Fasting - Limits your calorie intake by narrowing the amount of time you allow yourself to eat during the day.

OMAD - Limits your calorie intake by allowing you to eat one meal a day.

Weight Watchers - Limits your calorie intake by using a point system.

In the prior section *"Just because you can, doesn't mean you should,"* we reviewed that there are a lot of ways to lose weight.

3 Power Questions

Before starting on any plan I recommend you answer 3 questions:

1. Does this fit my eating profile?

2. Is it practical for my schedule/life?

3. What's my goal for time frame length/results from it?

Most people will focus on the result first and fall off track when it's not a fit for their daily life.

For example, you may want to try intermittent fasting, but your work/break schedule makes it unrealistic.

Don't swim upstream from the very start. Find something that is practical, fits for your desired goals, and go for it!

Why Diets Fail

So if all diets *can* work, why do we struggle so much with getting and staying healthy. Here's a quick list of the top reasons.

Expectations don't match reality. When someone expects to fully undo 10 years of bad eating habits in 10 weeks or even 10 days, there's going to be a disconnect.

Doesn't fit the lifestyle. Look deeper than the principles of any diet you want to follow. Take a look at your schedule, your eating preferences, and food that is readily available to you.

No exit strategy. If you're on a "rabbit" style eating plan, you'll need to pre-plan an end date and decide which plan you'll move to after that. Otherwise, you'll hit the wall and be tempted to splurge.

Helps with weight loss but you feel like crap. Either the calorie deficit is too much or you or you become low on a micronutrient from eliminating too many choices. The scale says lighter but you don't feel a bit healthier.

Section Two - Common Eating and Fitness Questions Explained

Over the years, we've assembled "how to" guides based off of common member questions. They're simple, straightforward, and have helped provide clarity during this journey.

So you'll find the information quickly, there's no extra fluff in these answers!

How to lose weight fastest and keep it off.

Adopt the rabbit habits around your personal calendar.

Make it practical to your tastes and preferences.

Plan a bridge into being a turtle around busy times like the holidays without going completely off track.

How to lose weight and keep it off.

Adopt the turtle's habits and stick to them year around. Throw in a few "rabbit" days after bigger indulgences to stay on track.

If a cheat meal turns into a cheat day, let it go. It happens and you're human. Re-calibrate with a good quality day the day after.

Another option is to plan ahead and have a "rabbit" day before you go into the event or get together.

How to stay the same and become fitter.

Adopt the baby turtle's habits and start building up "wins."

Use exercise to build lean muscle, increase your metabolism, and renew your energy. Similar to picking your eating profile, pick exercise that is practical for you to do on a regular basis.

There's a ton of mindset benefits with this approach.

If you were gaining weight slowly and are now staying the same and feeling great, that's one in the win column.

I'm sharing this truth to simply manage expectations so you stay on track. It will be a slower road for weight loss.

However, if you realize that upfront, you'll likely enjoy the many benefits you can build while being in this profile.

How to stay the same.

Eat relatively healthy meals most of the time.

Exercise sometimes throughout the year.

Most people gain weight every year, so staying the same can be a win for some!

This is a realistic place to be for people that bounce from exercise plan to exercise plan and diet to diet.

How to gain unwanted weight.

This is a tough truth that needs to be covered in case you find yourself landing in these habits.

You may get stuck in spectator mode, especially around holidays and vacations.

I've seen a trend in the fall of people going off track and gaining body fat. School starts for kids, and parents need time to adjust. Their exercise hits the back burner.

When they're ready, it's close to Thanksgiving with all the family obligations, so they put it off.

Then it's almost Christmas so it gets put off again until New Years.

Next it takes a few more weeks to get going again, so sometime around February we see a big uptick in people ready to kick butt...until the fall again.

How to get started without burning out.

Replace before you restrict.

This is a powerful concept I first read about from the folks at Precision Nutrition. They're right on the money with this suggestion.

Replace junk food with similar quantities of healthy food. Avoid counting calories and simply eat a lot of healthy food so you don't feel so restricted.

You'll get most of your results and when you hit a plateau, then, and only then, start worrying about the restriction.

And the little magic secret behind this approach is that it's tough to eat the same calories of healthy food. You'd have to eat nearly 10 bags of spinach to equal the same calories in an ice cream sundae.

You'll naturally start eating less and feeling fuller without even realizing it.

How to meal prep.

When I was a kid (that's how you know I'm getting old!), "meal prepping" was simply called "eating leftovers."

Most families over prepare their dinners and then have the leftovers during lunch the next day. It's a great system and I have 1 big tweak.

When you cook a healthy dinner, make a larger portion. Divide it up into single serving containers and store.

There's something psychological about opening the fridge and seeing your meal ready in a single serving tupperware versus crammed in a huge one.

You're more likely to grab and go if you took the 5 seconds to leverage this tip the evening before!

Meal prepping the big items will help you plan your grocery list, save hassle, and save money in the long run. You're less likely to have nothing ready and go out to dinner instead.

How to figure out why you aren't losing weight.

Give some honest thought to the following (I'm putting them in the order that I see them occur).

You haven't been patient. It took time to gain the weight and it won't go away in a few weeks. Stay the course and focus on non-scale victories to build momentum.

You have unrealistic expectations. This goes hand in hand with the reason above. It's also a primary purpose of going over the full eating profiles and game plan in this book. Managing expectations will be critical to your success.

You identified your profile incorrectly. You think you're eating like a turtle but the cheat meals add up. It's likely you're not in a calorie deficit overall and the pounds are sticking around.

You haven't been consistent enough. A few good days doesn't make a full plan. It's like a football team throwing a beautiful touchdown pass, then immediately giving up a kick return touchdown to go down 30-7.

Some of the above.

All of the above.

How to stay on track in the long term.

The best way is to not let moments that knock you off track, keep you off track. Slip ups happen and the guilt associated only "helps" if you bounce right back.

Spend less time worrying about perfecting a plan and more time figuring out how to stay consistent even when you don't want to.

I'll write it one more time to make sure you're set up for long term success.

Spend less time worrying about perfecting a plan and more time figuring out how to stay consistent even when you don't want to.

How to burn stubborn belly fat.

First, if we're talking exercise you'll want to do compound exercises like push ups, squats, etc. These exercises use multiple muscle groups and will burn more fat than isolation exercises like a simple bicep curl or crunch.

It's typically best to work with a pro so they can select what's best for your fitness level and health history.

Honestly, one of the best overall exercises is jokingly called plate pushes.

When you're sitting at the table, push the plate away from you when you're full.

If you're eating slowly, including protein, and getting your veggies in, you'll fill up and self regulate through a lot of the hurdles.

When you're doing your big picture exercises and eating right (with a dash of patience), the belly fat will start to shed.

How to understand carbs

We're going really basic on this one to just give the info that will help you on towards your goals.

Carbohydrates are a great energy source for your body. When they are digested and shuttled through your bloodstream, your body will prefer to burn these versus reaching into stubborn fat reserves.

You should eat them around times that you need energy, such as a workout. They'll give you a quick boost in case you feel like you're dragging.

If you want more, add in additional carbs on days where you have more intense training. For example, a sweet potato with dinner on a leg day.

Want fruit? Put it about 60 minutes before your workout to get the most out of the energy provided.

Can you do other things with high carb, low carb, and everything in between? Yes. Walk before you can run to help build habits. The basics above will get you on the right path and most of the way there. Once you reach a real plateau, then start tweaking things.

How to manage the "I'm so hungry" feeling

Ghrelin, a hormone that helps digestion gives you a lot of the "hungry" feeling.

By developing a pattern to always eat at a certain time, you created a cycle of feeling hungry at that time because your body is preparing for food digestion with ghrelin.

First, give any new eating plan a few weeks for your body to adjust. If you're replacing before you restrict, you're likely getting enough calories.

In as soon as a few days, the "I'm hungry" feeling that typically happens around your afternoon snack starts to dissipate.

How to control cravings.

The excellent book called "Power of Habit" explained Habit Loops and how to break them up successfully.

A typical craving lasts 15-20 minutes for reasons covered in the previous question.

Ever get so involved in something that you forget to eat dinner? Or you get on a task and you didn't even think about a snack?

You'll leverage the same concept, except this time it will be on purpose.

First, identify a "trouble" time of day that triggers a bad eating habit. For a lot of people it's night time. Parents get the kids to bed and finally have a few peaceful minutes to relax, so they reward themselves with some cheese and wine.

Instead, you need to find something that you also enjoy to replace the eating part of the habit.

Night time will inevitably come around so think ahead and build a list of active things you can do to get through it without making it a pure test of willpower.

Examples include:

- Work on a hobby

- Clear your inbox

- Journal or mind dump to clear your head

- Send a thoughtful text to a friend or relative

- Go for a bike ride

- Shoot some hoops in the driveway (my go to)

- Do a 10 minute follow-along YouTube video for something like Yoga

The more active you make your items, the better they will work. Often sitting still, like watching TV, is another trigger and makes it more challenging.

Take a minute to come up with a few of your own go-to solutions.

Plug and play when a craving approaches!

Frequently Asked Questions

When I first developed the eating profiles, they were shared in a workshop attended by around 100 gym members. Every attendee wrote down the answer to the following 2 questions on an index card:

1. What's going well with your eating and fitness?

2. What do you need more support on?

I collected all the cards so I'd be able to follow up with them and get the information in their hands after the workshop.

Many have already been answered in the previous "how to" section and there was a lot of duplicates as well.

Here are the major ones that I think will help you along the way.

How do I combine exercise and nutrition for weight loss?

As you've read in this book, there's a lot of different ways to approach eating based on your profile. Here's a few ways you can get it done.

If you're new to both diet and exercise, choose 1 as your "foundational habit." This is a habit that you can get done no matter how crazy the day gets. For most, it's 45-60 minutes of exercise. It's more controllable than a full day's eating plan.

For some it's something like eating a veggie with every meal.

Always do that habit--with no exceptions.

This let's you get over the guilty feeling and falling off when a few stressful days occur.

Another way is to start a new eating plan and moderate exercise so you're not burning out. If you're restricting in the kitchen, don't expect to be successful at a super aggressive new fitness program at the same time.

A third way is to go all in on exercise. Focus on growing stronger first. Soon you'll not want to "waste" those sessions by eating bad food, and it will be easier to buy into one of the eating profiles.

Exactly like the eating profiles, you'll need to select an approach that's a fit for you and go with it. There are lots of ways to get there, but there are also a lot of ways to let time pass and do nothing.

Choose one path and if you want to switch it later, you'll have the freedom to do so by knowing you'll still get to your results.

How do I grocery shop better?

Great question! I've screwed this one up a lot by going to the store hungry, browsing the aisles to see what speaks to me, and ending up making poor choices.

The best grocery shopping days have been when there is a meal plan in place.

Take your eating profile, look at the recipe guides provided later on in this book, and plan out your meals. If you have a family, add in the basics of what they'd like too.

Get your veggies and proteins first. They're the base of your meals and should be the base of your grocery shopping too. If you are pressed for time or the store gets packed, you'll already have these fundamentals done.

Next add in the other items on your list and get out of there!

Like with weight loss, be patient with yourself. After a few weeks, you'll have a good grasp of how much to pick up each trip to have a successful week.

Here's an extreme option for someone that is single and needs quick weight loss. I read about a person online that cleaned out all of his cupboards. The temptation was too great. Instead, he walked the miles to the grocery story each morning, bought just enough for the day, and walked home.

He lost an amazing amount of weight by trying something a bit different.

It's likely your approach will fall somewhere between these extremes based on family needs and personal tastes.

When should I eat?

Over the last 15 or so years, the thought was that 6 smaller meals a day would boost your metabolism. Studies since have shown that it doesn't make much of a difference as long as the total consumption is the same.

So the short answer is whenever you want as long as it follows your eating profile.

If you aren't hungry in the morning and want to push back more food to around an afternoon workout, you're free to do so.

If you prefer the smaller meals and lots of variety, go for it.

I've even seen people only eat one large meal a day. In the early 2000s I was coaching football with an older gentleman that had lost 60 lbs and kept it off for the better part of two decades.

He explained that he only ate dinner. If he was hungry, he'd have a small piece of fruit or something midday. Other than that, he had been feeling great, lost weight, and impressed doctors by only eating his one meal for nearly 20 years.

They'll all work as long as you choose what's a fit for you and stick to the overall plan.

The total over the course of the full day will matter more for you than minute by minute.

How much protein should I eat?

The recommended daily allowance (RDA) to avoid a protein deficiency is .36 grams per body lb.

However, staying out of a deficiency and being at the optimal amount are very different things. Let's put it this way. Getting only the RDA is like earning a 65 in high school math class. Sure, you'll barely pass, but it's not the best situation.

According to the most recent school of thought, .7 to .8 grams per body lb will be better for a person that is engaged in daily exercise.

You can avoid a lot of kitchen math by sticking to the guidelines recommended in the eating profiles. Every meal contains a protein source already.

Another way to simplify it is by using the palm of your hand. If you're a larger adult, you'd have 2 palm sized portions with each meal. Otherwise, 1 palm sized protein portion will be a good starting point.

Simplifying will get you in the game without too much friction. I always recommend tracking your results to see if you're on the right path.

We use the Inbody 570 (and there are other medical grade body composition machines just as good). If you see skeletal muscle mass dropping on repeat scans over a 4-6 weeks, it would be time to look at your protein intake, total calories, and exercise intensity.

If things are aligned on each test, then keep up the simple methods.

If things fall off, then make adjustments from there.

But you can never make in-game adjustments if you're still on the sidelines.

How do I find the motivation to get started?

I've never been a big "rah rah" person, although finding a few motivational speeches may help you get the ball rolling.

Instead, I recommend two strategies.

First, have a plan and develop realistic expectations. Follow the steps in the quick start guide in the next section, choose your eating profile, and be confident in the strategy.

I need to emphasize this one more time. The realistic expectations are absolutely critical and I reference them throughout this book. You may find motivation in a quick results diet plan, but it will evaporate at the very first negative result or speed bump along the way.

Second, harness your "why power." It's a term we use at Synergy and have a full wall dedicated to it at each of our locations.

Ask yourself, "Why is this important for me to accomplish?"

Write down that answer, for example, "to feel better."

Don't stop there. Ask, "Why is that important to me?" To continue our example, "Why is feeling better important to me?"

Maybe it's "because I have low energy at home and I don't like that."

"Why is having more energy at home important to me?"

"Because I want to play with my kids more and have them see me as a healthy person."

Then you repeat asking and answering until you have a more powerful reply. Initially it may be to feel better, which is a great motivator to get started.

After peeling back the layers, it may also be because you want to be a role model for your kids and set them up with healthy habits even though you didn't have that luxury growing up.

It usually takes 4-7 rounds of asking "why" and you'll have different levels of answers. All are important and all can keep you on track even when you don't want to do it.

Answer to every recipe question

The recipe section in this book will help get you thinking of ideas. Maybe there are 1-2 that you end up using but maybe not. My tastes are likely different than yours.

I don't like fancy prepared meals and would prefer to have quiet time to eat something plain. I prioritize ease and speed over taste. So my personal examples may not be a fit for you.

Here's how to solve every recipe question.

1. Look at your eating profile.

2. Think of food items that you like and that fit within that profile.

3. Do an internet search for recipes with those ideas.

4. Choose one and try it.

Here's a few search terms to help you get started:

- Quick protein snacks - 85.5 million

- Protein and veggie meal ideas - 143 million

- Protein family meal - 163 million (and I'm making one of the results tonight!)

- Ideas to eat more vegetables - 160 million

- Veggie snack ideas - 158 million

- Veggie snack ideas for work - 114 million

You can see I kept trying longer keyword phrases to stump Google. Nope, I couldn't do it! Every search had great ideas within the very first two pages.

And the cool part is, you don't have to do these searches more than a couple of times to find a few "go to" ideas that are a fit for you.

Your eating profile will provide clarity to your overall strategy. Now you have the knowledge to plug and play recipes based on your personal tastes, preferences, and schedule.

Quick Start Guide

Early on in this book, I used an analogy about a football game. Most people look for tips and tricks, aka "the plays," but never develop the big picture game plan.

After reading this, you have the "playbook" to get into the game and starting putting up wins. Here's the guide.

How To Implement This Book.

1. Read the eating profiles and identify where you are today.

2. Look at a calendar. Plan which eating profile you'll use during which dates.

3. Remove obstacles. This includes:

•   Looking at the recipe guide or do an internet search based on your tastes to find "plays" that will work for you.

•   Setting realistic expectations.

•   Writing down your "why power."

•   Identifying times of day that you fall off and re-read the question, "How to control cravings."

4. Start

5. When you hit a roadblock, refer to the section "How to figure out why you aren't losing weight."

6. Re-identify any new roadblocks.*

7. Keep going, you can do this!

8. Repeat steps 5-8.

* Roadblocks will come up along the way. It's very common. It's like getting in a football game and all of a sudden the other team sets up in a way that you never expected.

It might sound silly, but you wouldn't expect a professional football team to line up, look across the ball, see something different, and run off the field and quit in a panic.

You'll need to adjust your strategy and you'll be perfectly fine.

The biggest one I hear is that, "I got bored/confused by not enough variety in my food choices."

The tough truth is that that is a very solvable roadblock.

Looking deeper it's more likely that you're losing momentum overall, the eating strategies aren't habits yet, and this happens to be an easy excuse to get out.

A Google search for "healthy protein recipes" just produced 86.6 million results. Finding something you like and solving this roadblock is just a few clicks away.

Don't let a few hiccups define your entire eating plan. Forgive any slip-ups fast. You're only 1 meal away from being right back on track.

Rabbit Habit Worksheet

If you've opted for rabbit habits, focus on these habits. Place a check mark in each box as you successfully complete each day.

Habits	Day 1	Day 2	Day 3	Day 4	Day 5	Day 6	Day 7
Vegetables with every meal							
Lean protein source with every meal							
No alcohol							
60 min of exercise or activity							
Full night's sleep							

Re-create this chart and deploy for each week you plan on sticking with the rabbit habits. Remember, weekends count too!

Turtle Habit Worksheet

If you've opted for turtle habits, focus on these habits. Place a check mark in each box as you successfully complete each day.

Habits	Day 1	Day 2	Day 3	Day 4	Day 5	Day 6	Day 7
At least 2 out of 3 meals contain vegetables and a protein							
Two or less cheat meals per week							
At least 60 minutes of exercise 3 times per week							
Put carb intake around exercise (like fruit)							
Full night's sleep							

Re-create this chart and deploy for each week you plan on sticking with the turtle habits. Remember, weekends count too!

Baby Turtle Habit Worksheet

If you've opted for baby turtle habits, focus on these habits. Place a check mark in each box as you successfully complete each day.

Habits	Day 1	Day 2	Day 3	Day 4	Day 5	Day 6	Day 7
Chews slowly to allow body to feel full							
Eats at least 1 vegetable a day							
Focuses on replacing before restricting							
Exercises at least twice a week and is active outside workouts							
Gets a full night's sleep most of the time.							

Re-create this chart and deploy for each week you plan on sticking with the baby turtle habits. Remember, weekends count too!

Rabbit Recipe Examples

Chorizo Egg Muffins

3.5oz Spanish chorizo or pepperoni

3.5oz chopped fresh kale

6 large eggs

1c unsweetened pumpkin puree

Salt and pepper

Optional: 1/2c grated cheddar cheese

Optional: sriracha sauce, greens, sliced avocado

Pre heat oven to 360. Dice the chorizo and place on a hot dry pan. Cook for 1-2 minutes to release the juices and crisp it up. Add kale and cook 5-7 minutes covered. Remove from heat and set aside.

Crack eggs into bowl and mix with pumpkin puree. Add the chorizo and kale. Season with salt and pepper, mix until combined. Add grated cheese (if using)

Spoon mixture into muffin tray (silicone trays work best) distribute evenly between 10 muffin cups. Bake for 20-25 minutes and set aside to cool slightly before serving. Serve with sriracha sauce, greens or sliced avocado if desired. Store in fridge in air tight container for up to 5 days.

Sweet Potato Hash

3 large sweet potatoes, peeled and chopped

2 bell peppers, chopped

1 large onion, chopped

3 cloves garlic, minced

3 tbs extra-virgin olive oil

Kosher salt

ground black pepper

1/4 tsp paprika

3 sprigs rosemary

Freshly chopped chives, for garnish

Preheat oven to 425°. On a large rimmed baking sheet, toss sweet potatoes with bell peppers, onion, garlic, and oil. Season with salt, pepper, and paprika. Scatter rosemary on top. Bake until sweet potatoes are crispy on the outside and soft on the inside, about 45 minutes, shaking the pan halfway through.

Garnish with chives to serve.

Bell Pepper Eggs

1 bell pepper, sliced into 1/4" rings

6 eggs

salt

ground black peppers

2 tbs chopped chives

2 tbs chopped parsley

Heat a nonstick skillet over medium heat, and grease lightly with cooking spray. Place a bell pepper ring in the skillet, then sauté for two minutes. Flip the ring, then crack an egg in the middle. Season with salt and pepper, then cook until the egg is cooked to your liking, 2 to 4 minutes. Repeat with the other eggs, then garnish with chives and parsley.

Buffalo Chicken Salad in a Jar

Buffalo Dressing:

1/4c mayonnaise

3tbs Sriracha sauce

¼ tsp Paprika

¼ tsp garlic powder

¼ tsp onion powder

Salt and pepper

2c diced cooked chicken

Salad:

1 medium avocado

1tbs fresh lemon juice

Optional: 1/3 c crumbled blue cheese

2 medium celery stalks sliced

1 small red onion sliced

4c mixed salad greens

To make the dressing, add all of the ingredients in a bowl. Mix until well combined, then add cooked chicken and mix again.

To make salad, halve peel and dice the avocado. Squeeze lemon juice over avocado to prevent it from browning. To assemble the salad, divide the dressed chicken between two 1 qt jars with wide mouths. Add a layer of blue cheese (if using) to each jar, followed by the celery, red onion, diced avocado and salad greens. When ready to serve tip the salad over into a serving bowl so the dressing covers the greens. Or, simply shake the jar, keeping the lid closed, and then eat the salad right from the jar. Store in sealed jar in the fridge for up to 3 days.

Turkey Mozzarella Roll-Ups

Thinly-sliced turkey stands in for the "tortilla" in these super-simple cheese wraps. Switch up the cheese throughout the week — we especially like cheddar, provolone, and dill Havarti.

Roll up 3 slices of deli turkey, with 3 slices of cheese

(Optional) Pack with: 1/2 avocado, cucumber slices

Chicken Sausage

Pre-cooked chicken sausage is a fast and easy choice for a fast and easy lunch. It comes in a huge variety of flavors (think: spicy andouille and Italian herb) so try new types throughout the week.

Just pick up a package of cooked chicken sausage, slice one, and pack it.

Pack with: Guacamole, radishes, French onion dip, almonds

Hot Beef and Broccoli Salad

1lb beef sirloin steak or stir fry meat

½ tsp salt

¼ tsp black pepper

2 tsp lemon zest

6tbs lemon garlic dressing

3c broccoli florets

1 large orange or red bell pepper thinly sliced

1 9oz package spring mix/baby spinach

1/4c fresh chives

Thinly slice the meat across the grain into bite size pieces and season both sides with the salt, pepper and lemon zest. In a medium bowl, toss the meat with 2 tbs of the dressing

In a large bowl, combine the broccoli, bell pepper and 3 tbs of the dressing. Toss to coat

In a large skillet, cook the broccoli and bell pepper over medium-high heat, stirring, for 3 minutes. Return the vegetables to the large bowl. Add the meat to the hot skillet and cook stirring until slightly pink in center, 1-2 minutes. Add the vegetables to the skillet and stir to combine with the meat.

In large bowl toss the greens with the remaining 1 tbs of dressing. Serve the meat and vegetables over the greens. Sprinkle the salad with the snipped chives.

Thai Chicken and Brussel Sprout Skillet

4 tbs extra virgin olive oil

1lb boneless skinless chicken thinly sliced

½ tsp salt

2 9-10oz bags of shaved brussels sprouts

1c shredded carrots

2 tbs chopped shallots

1/2c Asian citrus dressing

Sriracha

In an extra-large skillet heat 2 tbs of the olive oil over medium heat. Add the chicken and cook, stirring occasionally for 3 minutes. Sprinkle the chicken with the salt. Add the remaining 2 tbs olive oil to the skillet, then the brussels sprouts, carrots and shallots. Cook, stirring occasionally until the sprouts are tender and lightly browned, 5-8 minutes. Add the dressing and heat through, about 1 minute. Serve with sriracha.

Lemon Garlic Shrimp and Veggies

1 tbs olive oil

1 medium zucchini, trimmed, halved length wise and cut into half moons

1 medium red bell pepper, cut into thin strips

1 lb peeled and deveined extra-large shrimp

3 cloves garlic minced

¼ ghee

¼ c fresh lemon juice

½ tsp salt

¼ tsp black pepper

1 16oz package cauliflower crumbles

¼ c chopped fresh parsley

Heat the olive oil in a large skillet over medium high heat. Add the zucchini and pepper strips and cook stirring occasionally for 3 minutes. Add the shrimp and garlic and cook, turning the shrimp and stirring the vegetables once, until the shrimp are opaque, 5-6 minutes. Transfer the shrimp mixture to a bowl and cover to keep warm.

To make lemon pan sauce, reduce the heat to medium and melt the ghee in the skillet. Add the lemon juice, salt and black pepper, bring to a boil and whisk until smooth.

Meanwhile cook cauliflower crumbles according to package directions.

Spoon the shrimp and vegetables over the cauliflower, drizzle with the lemon sauce, sprinkle with parsley if desired and serve.

Crunchy Chile-Lime Nuts

1c walnuts

1c pecans

1c almonds

1c macadamia nuts

1tsp salt

½ tsp ground cumin

½ tsp paprika

¼ tsp cayenne pepper

¼ tsp black pepper

Optional: 1tbs erythritol or swerve

1tbs lime juice

2 tbs melted virgin coconut oil or ghee

Pre-heat oven to 350. Place all ingredients in a mixing bowl and mix until all ingredients are combined and nuts are well coated. Spread mixture in a single layer on a baking sheet lined with parchment paper. Roast for 8-12 minutes mixing the nuts with a spatula half way through. Remove from oven and let cool. Store in airtight container

Turtle Recipe Examples

Blissful Blueberry Smoothie

1 ½ c of fresh or frozen blueberries

½ c of non-dairy vanilla yogurt

¼ c rolled oats (optional)

2 c of almond milk

Optional: 2-4 ice cubes

Optional: 1 scoop of protein powder

Place all ingredients in a blender and blend on high until smooth and frothy.

** Recipe can be made gluten free using gluten free oats

Crockpot Apple Cinnamon Steel-cut Oatmeal

2 c of steel-cut oats

4 c of water

5 c of milk (skim, almond milk, etc.)

1 large honey crisp apple cut into ½ inch pieces

1 tsp cinnamon

1 tsp vanilla

½ tsp sea salt

Combine all ingredients in the slow-cooker and cook on LOW overnight, 7-8 hrs.

Taco Salad in a Jar

2 tbs extra-virgin olive oil

1 lb ground turkey

kosher salt

1 tbs Taco Seasoning

1 15-oz can black beans, rinsed and warmed

2 c frozen corn, thawed and warmed

1 head romaine, chopped

1 c shredded pepper Jack cheese

1 c diced tomatoes

In a large skillet, heat oil over medium-high heat. Add turkey and season with salt and taco seasoning. Cook, breaking up with the back of a wooden spoon or spatula, until deeply golden and cooked through, 8 to 10 minutes. Set aside and let cool 5 minutes.

Among six mason jars, layer ground turkey, black beans, corn, romaine, cheese, and tomatoes.

Spinach Salad

5 oz fresh spinach

1 apple, such as Fuji, thinly sliced

1/3 c crumbled feta

1/4 red onion, thinly sliced

1/4 c sliced almonds, toasted

Dressing

1/3 c olive oil

3 tbs red wine vinegar

1 clove garlic, minced

2 tsp dijon mustard

Kosher salt

Freshly ground black pepper

Combine all salad ingredients in a large bowl. Add dressing, toss to combine, and serve immediately.

Spicy Grilled Shrimp with Pineapple Sauce

1 lb large shrimp, cooked, deveined

6 grilling skewers

2 tbs coconut oil or butter

¼ tsp cayenne powder

½ tsp crushed red pepper

1 lime

Optional: 2 tbs fresh cilantro (optional)

6 grape tomatoes minced

3/4 cup pineapple minced

Preheat the grill to about 350 degrees (or medium-high heat). Fully thaw the shrimp and place about 4-5 shrimp on each skewer. Mix the oil/butter and cayenne powder together, then coat each shrimp skewer. Grill on each side for about 3-5 minutes or until opaque.

Mix the minced pineapple and minced tomatoes together to create the salsa. Top each shrimp skewer with crushed red pepper, fresh lime juice, cilantro, and pineapple salsa.

Serve and enjoy!

Chicken Broccoli Pasta Casserole

3 c almond milk

½ c chicken broth

½ c cashew butter

2 tbs almond flour

8 oz. gluten-free spiral pasta

1 large broccoli head (about 3 c florets)

2 cooked chicken breasts, cubed

¼ tsp salt

½ tsp pepper

Optional: 2 tbs crushed walnuts

Optional: ¼ c cheese

Preheat oven to 350 degrees. Mix the almond milk, chicken broth, cashew butter, and almond flour together. Set aside.

Place the dry pasta in the bottom of a casserole dish. Layer the broccoli on top of the pasta. Pour 3/4 of the almond milk mixture over the pasta and broccoli. Bake for about 15 minutes (or until pasta is soft).

Remove the pan from the oven and add the chicken. Add the salt and pepper. Pour the remaining almond milk mixture over the casserole and add optional walnuts and cheese.

Bake for another 10-15 minutes (or until everything is hot). Serve and enjoy!

Lemon-Dijon Pork Sheet Pan Dinner

4 tsp Dijon mustard

2 tsp grated lemon zest

1 garlic clove, minced

½ tsp salt

2 tbs canola oil

1-1/2 lbs sweet potatoes (about 3 medium), cut into 1/2-inch cubes

1 lb fresh Brussels sprouts (about 4 c), quartered

4 boneless pork loin chops (6 oz each)

Optional: Coarsely ground pepper

Preheat oven to 425°. In a large bowl, mix first 4 ingredients; gradually whisk in oil. Remove 1 tablespoon mixture for brushing pork. Add vegetables to remaining mixture; toss to coat.

Place pork chops and vegetables in a 15x10x1-in. pan coated with cooking spray. Brush chops with reserved mustard mixture. Roast 10 minutes.

Turn chops and stir vegetables; roast until a thermometer inserted in pork reads 145° and vegetables are tender, 10-15 minutes longer. If desired, sprinkle with pepper. Let stand 5 minutes before serving.

Baby Turtle Recipe Examples

Sweet Rice and Fruit

3 c cooked rice

1 c plain yogurt

1 -2 bananas sliced

2 tbs honey or maple syrup

Freshly squeezed lemon or orange juice

Optional: 2 tbs nut butter (stirred into yogurt)

Add splash of water to the rice and warm in sauté pan over medium-high heat. Divide rice onto two plates. Top with yogurt and banana slices and drizzle with honey and citrus juice. Add salt to taste.

Scrambled Egg Tacos

Eggs

Soft taco shells

Optional: Cheese

Optional: Salsa

Optional: Frank's Red Hot

Scramble eggs Place in a "taco" soft shell. Add in desired optional items cheese, salsa, or frank's red hot

Peanut Butter Banana Roll Up

Natural Peanut Butter

Banana cut into slices

Wrap

Spread natural peanut butter on a wrap. Thinly slice a banana and place the slices on the peanut butter Start at one end and roll it up.

Chocolate Yogurt

Plain Greek yogurt

½ - ¾ scoop of chocolate protein powder

Whole Oats

Optional: Jelly or Jam

Mix together: chocolate protein powder and plain Greek yogurt - Sprinkle in a few whole oats - Spoonful of jelly or jam (for added sweetness) That will have the added sugar, but at least you can control the portion size better

Avocado Tuna Salad

1 3 oz pouch Albacore Tuna, no salt added

1 ripe avocado

1 tbs minced red onion

1 tsp minced jalapeno

½ tsp kosher salt

1 lime (juice of)

¼ tsp garlic powder

In a mixing bowl, mash the avocado with the salt, lime juice and garlic powder. Mix in the jalapeno, onion, and cilantro until well combined. Add in the tuna and mix until tuna is evenly distributed. Serve on a sandwich, in a wrap, in a lettuce wrap, on crackers or alone.

Tomato Avocado Bagelwiches

1 everything bagel

2 tbs veggie cream cheese

1 heirloom tomato sliced

½ avocado sliced

1 pinch smoked sea salt

1 tbs chopped chives

1 drizzle extra virgin olive oil

1 handful spicy microgreens

Spread the cream cheese on one or both sides of the bagel. Add the tomatoes on one side and the avocado on the other. Sprinkle both with smoked salt, the chives and then drizzle with olive oil. Add the microgreens on top, then sandwich the bagel together.

Egg Salad

6 hard-boiled eggs peeled and chopped

2 ½ tbs plain greek yogurt

1 ½ tbs mayonnaise

1 ½ tbs dill pickle juice

2 tsp sweet relish

1 tsp dijon mustard

3 tbss freshly snipped chives plus extra for topping

¼ tsp salt

¼ tsp pepper

1/8 tsp smoked paprika

Optional: butter lettuce

Optional: pickled onions

Optional: grainy bread toasted

Optional: smoked sea salt for sprinkling

To make the salad, place the chopped hard-boiled eggs in a bowl. I usually add everything to the egg bowl, but if desired, you can whisk it up first! Stir together the yogurt, mayo, pickle juice, relish and mustard. Gently toss the eggs in the mixture. Fold in the chives, salt, pepper and paprika.

Place a piece of butter lettuce on toast, top it with the salad and then top it with pickled onions and smoked sea salt!

Instapot Sweet and Sour Chicken

1 lb boneless, skinless chicken breasts, cut into 1-inch chunks

½ tbs canola oil

1 onion, diced into 1-inch chunks

1 red pepper, cut into 1-inch chunks

1 yellow pepper, cut into 1-inch chunks

1 cup fresh pineapple, cut into 1-inch chunks

1 tbs minced garlic

½ c chicken stock or water

½ c apricot all fruit jam

2 tbs soy sauce

¼ c rice wine vinegar

1 tbs cornstarch

Turn Instant Pot function to sauté and heat the oil. Add chicken and sauté just until lightly browned on all sides--about 2 minutes.

Add remaining ingredients (except for cornstarch) to Instant Pot and thoroughly stir. Close Instant Pot and cook on high pressure for 5 minutes (under poultry setting if your pot has this setting). Be sure to seal the vent.

Once chicken has cooked, do a quick release method after 5 minutes. Turn Instant Pot back to sauté and add the cornstarch that has been mixed with 1 tablespoon water back into the Instant Pot. Bring to a boil and let sauce thicken.

Healthy Homemade Hamburger Helper Skillet

1 lb ground sirloin or turkey

1 6 oz can of tomato paste

1 tsp paprika

1 tsp onion powder

1 tsp garlic powder

1 tsp salt

½ tsp freshly ground black pepper

1 8 oz can of tomato sauce

3 ½ c MSG free low-sodium beef broth

2 c dried whole wheat elbow macaroni noodles

1 tsp Worchester sauce

Heat a large skillet over medium-high heat. Add in the meat and brown up, breaking up into small pieces. Once meat is cooked, drain off any fat and return to heat.

Add tomato paste and seasonings. Cook for 2 minutes to develop flavor. Add in tomato sauce and beef broth and bring to a boil.

Add in noodles and turn down to medium heat. Cook for 10-12 minutes, stirring occasionally, or until noodles cooked through and sauce is absorbed. Stir in Worchester sauce and serve.

Tortellini Broth Bowl

1 16 oz package fresh cheese tortellini

1 5 oz package fresh spinach

1 pint heirloom grape tomatoes, sliced in quarters

1 clove garlic minced

2 c vegetable stock

½ c dry white wine or additional stock

juice of 1 lemon

2 sprigs fresh thyme

¼ c panko bread crumbs

1 tsp olive oil

salt and pepper to taste

Parmesan cheese for serving

Prepare the tortellini according to package directions. While tortellini is cooking, bring the chicken stock, wine, 1 spring of thyme and garlic to a boil. Reduce heat and simmer for 10 minutes. Add in juice of fresh lemon juice at end of cooking.

Heat the olive oil in a small skillet over medium heat. Add bread crumbs and remaining sprig of thyme-- leaves chopped up. Toast until crumbs are golden brown, bout 2-3 minutes.

Evenly divide spinach and tomatoes and tortellini between 4 bowls. Ladle broth over each bowl. Sprinkle bread crumb mixture of each bowl and finish

with freshly grated Parmesan. Season with salt and
pepper and serve immediately

Conclusion

I'm excited for you to get started with your new eating strategies, plans, and tactics. It is my sincere hope that you've received value from reading this book.

If you'd like additional guidance, we're here to help.

Here's how:

1. Talk to us on the phone. Want to see if Synergy is the right fit for you? Want to talk to someone that cares about your success and can point you in the right direction towards it? We can help.

Just email joe@synergyfitnessteam.com with "CALL" in the subject and your number in the email. We'll get right back to you.

2. Book a free session. We'll evaluate your goals and fitness level first. From there, you'll get our expert advice on how to achieve your goals and be guided through a 60 minute session that is a good fit for you.

Just email joe@synergyfitnessteam.com with "FREE TRIAL" we'll get right back to you.

3. Risk-free 30-Day Jumpstart. If you've seen enough of our members incredible results and you're ready to get started, our 30 Day Jumpstart is the perfect fit. You'll get the full Synergy Experience, designed to get you on the path to a longer, healthier and happier life!

Just email joe@synergyfitnessteam.com with "JUMPSTART" in the subject line and we'll get right back to you.